DASH DIET
FOR BEGINNERS

BONUS INCLUDED
35 TOP DASH DIET RECIPES!

VALERIE CHILDS

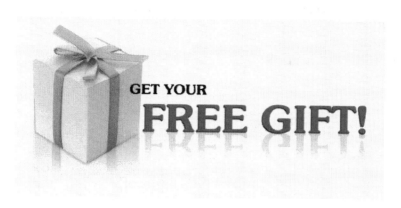

GET YOUR

FREE GIFT!

WAIT! – DO YOU LIKE FREE BOOKS?

My **FREE Gift** to You!! As a way to say **Thank You** for downloading my book, I'd like to offer you more **FREE BOOKS!** Each time we release a NEW book, we offer it first to a small number of people as a test - drive. Because of your commitment here in downloading my book, I'd love for you to be a part of this group. You can join easily here → http://rapidslimdown.com/

CONTENTS

INTRODUCTION

M y health was still of concern, physically, though mentally I had done laps around myself. My nutrition was initially able to regain my body and confidence and steer clear from the doom of my own death bed. My story is not extraordinary, but it certainly shows the major shift to self realization and treating my body as a temple with the types of food that I put into it.

As I had always been a naysayer of dieting and a harsh critic to those who needed it, I found myself perusing many of the nutritional approaches, often categorized as diets. But it was not until I tried many of the less than stellar ones, that I realized what I needed was a lifestyle approach in order to keep the weight off and maintain a healthy body image. I tried the low carb versions of diets, such as Atkins, Mediterranean, and South Beach. I was drawn to them based on the appeal of quick results, not by the value of their nutritional approach. I had planned for the wedding in one year, and I needed some major results, as I was more overweight than I had ever been, despite my healthier lifestyle.

The low carb diets were great at taking weight off, but they generally did not allow me to utilize my wide range of tastes in food. This became my downfall. After a successful bout at 30 pounds, which I was able to take off in a mean two months, eating bacon wrapped scallops, shrimp and steak, I was delighted in the ability for ketosis to do its magic. But the honeymoon phase to the marriage of meat did not seem to last, and my hankering for sugar and carbs crept in, just as quickly as the summer died off. The holidays were the worst and put an end to my carb cutting ways. I had gained almost all of the weight back, to my dismay.

Low fat diets seemed initially appealing as the best solution in my mind, but I found out from friends who had dealt with dieting all their life, that this was a gimmick of the 80s and 90s. The more modern theory on weight loss seemed to come to terms with the fact that low fat was not successful or satisfying. The packaged food industry seemed to have profited from this hype. While a lower fat intake can always be healthier, I learned that fats can also be good for you. I increased healthy fats and branched out to new foods. Avocados were a new favorite, as was coconut oil and ghee in Indian food. Other types of diets, like weight watchers, which are raved by so many did not seem to work for me simply due to the counting and accountability to strangers. My introverted personality seemed to stay with me in all that I seemed to have lost. Groups and meetings where I had to weigh in on a scale did not suit well for me.

Despite the fact that this next trial seems like a great but cheesy testimonial for a major drug company, it is not. It does resemble the ramblings of a tried and true and ecstatic customer of a product, but it is not something that can be bought. It does seem very ironic that my statement regarding this begins with the phrase, "I spoke to my doctor about the trials and tribulations of my disease and he recommended this." Despite those ironies, it is sheer honesty and joy that I beam with now. I am not a paid and walking advertisement for a pharmaceutical company, and I am not a salesperson for anything, although that happened to be my previous career. I found a solution to weight loss, heart disease, general health, and happiness for life.

My doctor offered the initial suggestion which has kick started a passion in me to tell all that I know of the benefits regarding the lifestyle change, also dubbed as a diet, known as DASH. It is not some product line for Kim Kardashian and it is not some dashingly quick way to shed pounds unrealistically. It is dubbed DASH for the acronym in its nomenclature. It stands for Dietary Approaches to Stop Hypertension and the National Heart, Lung, and Blood Institute in the United States created it as an intention of not being a fad diet for the face of a celebrity, but rather being the healthy lifestyle choice as recommended.

If you are seeking a solution to a vanity obsessed reason to lose weight, you are not alone. This was indeed my own poor health and poorer mindset a mere few years ago. My life had no time for concern with the health stakes of poor lifestyle choices. It was just like the average American woman, overweight and yet also weight-obsessed! To be out of control and yet believing yourself to be in control, with each new trendy diet, fitness routine, or smart phone application to reel in your weight gain. The paradox continues to keep women unhealthy and unable to realize their best health potential. So, if this is you, then you must realize this is your saving grace. This approach to life in a way that is not calorie obsessed nor body obsessed; it is a subtle approach of being body conscious and calorie conscious. It is gentle and perfect for those who like myself, speculated on the reasons why diets fail, for the simple fact that eating less is indeed part of the problem. But it teaches you that it is not the entire and whole problem. Eating is not the sole reason for weight gain or poor health and hypertension. While it does have an effect, there is much more to the problem.

CHAPTER 1

WHAT IS THE DASH DIET?

Although the emergence of the DASH Diet in pop culture is just now seeming to take flight, it is not something at all which is new. It was established over a decade ago, with the first actual references to it being in 2002. Dr. Oz refers to it as "The Little Diet That Could" on his popular television show, claiming it to be the most famous diet for three years in a row. Despite its trendy ways, it is the number one overall diet, three years running, and will help you drop pounds in just weeks, but also something that you will be able to stick to easily for life. It lowers cholesterol and increases antibodies against cancer. There's more research on this diet, according to Doctor and Professor Caroline Aprovian, than any other diet ever created. It is completely backed by the medical community, as a whole, which is hard to be said about all diets. And that is among thousands! It is all about portion control combined with the correct whole foods, and it makes it such an appeal. It was created by the government health agency known as the *National Heart, Lung and Blood Institution* despite its popularity running amuck amidst many third party sellers. It is not something you need to pay anyone for, as a little common sense and basic guidelines listed on various credible websites will give you. (Dr. Oz, 2013) The reason it was created could be speculated that the rising concern for women and heart disease had been developing as a major cause of premature death in the United States. It happens to affect women, and women are indeed followers of dieting trends, more so than are men.

CHAPTER 2

WHY WAS THE DASH DIET CREATED?

The diet, which is known to some, like myself, as a complete transformation, manifesto, and lifestyle change is an acronym which stands for "Dietary Approach to Stop Hypertension." Its primary purpose is to lower sodium consumption and also to reduce the pandemic of hypertension in many people's health charts. A lifestyle predisposed by sodium consumption and also mere family history can affect this hypertension. This seemed to be a necessary cause of creating a need to educate and guide the public consumer and citizen to make wiser health decisions concerning their diet and consumption of foods. A contender in the field of the dash diet is the website, dashdiet.org, which makes this statement as to the effects:

The DASH diet helps to lower blood pressure by providing more key nutrients, such as potassium, calcium, and magnesium, all of which are associated with lower blood pressure. These key nutrients are boosted by including more fruits, vegetables, and low-fat or nonfat dairy in your daily diet. Some people see additional benefits by lowering sodium or salt in their diet. Our book includes additional lifestyle changes to lower blood pressure, such as weight loss, exercise, smoking cessation, and moderation of alcohol intake.

CHAPTER 3

CHARACTERISTICS OF THE DASH DIET:

This diet or lifestyle is composed of common sense nutrition, but in a way that is more regimented, with guidelines and health assessments based on age groups and sex. It is rich in fruits, vegetables, whole grains, and low fat dairy food stuff. It is not limited to any food groups and encompasses the importance of a well balanced and well rounded diet. This aspect of it makes it much easier and enjoyable to the average person as many diets are very restrictive to types of food. It is a diet which includes meal plans that allow meat, fish, poultry, nuts, and beans. The ever growing industry of processed foods may take a blow if the general public catches onto its poor affect on the body and mind. The DASH Diet is limiting only on the processed foods, sugar, artificial sugar, red meat, and added and unnecessary fats. It is one of the few diets recommended by the United States Department of Agriculture.

CHAPTER 4

WHY THE DASH DIET IS THE BEST APPROACH TO HEALTH AND WEIGHT LOSS?

1.   EASY TO FOLLOW

In a convenient world, it is no wonder that our diets must fit the same expectation. This approach to dieting is extremely uncomplicated and quite frankly so very simple and commonsensical. But we do know that in this modern age, people are lacking quite a bit of that. Due to our excess lifestyles, we have often forgotten the basics in simple pleasures, such as food and proper nutrition. Our bodies are able to heal themselves and to bounce back from whatever we have done to them. That itself is a miracle. We should honor our bodies with this notion.

If people can keep a general idea of the main food groups, being easy to follow ones, like fresh whole fruit, fresh whole vegetables, lean proteins. Simple as that—a balanced diet with back to basics approach.

2. NUTRITIOUS

No major food groups are boycotted in this diet which is a rarity in the diet world. It is a simple yet well rounded and wholly balanced nutritional lifestyle which lends to the fact that all things—and in this case, foods—in moderation, which is an excellent motto to live by.

3. SAFE

The fact that the research is there, the medical field will claim this diet to fame, before any other celebrity face will. It is trust of the consumer, not being sold on something, but rather being given an honest medical opinion on the matter as importance as their health and overall wellbeing.

4. EFFECTIVE FOR SHORT & LONG TERM WEIGHT LOSS

While the diet was created for the simple hope and successful conclusion to reduce hypertension, the effective weight loss is not something to be looked at lightly. It is a sure sign that proper health goes hand in hand with ideal body weight, less health issues, and a slimmer physique.

5. HELPS FIGHT DIABETES AND HEALTH DISEASE

The other unforeseen aspect of utilizing the DASH diet is in the successful testimonials and medical research found in the Diabetes and Health Diseases. It is an added bonus, as if the others weren't already enough.

CHAPTER 5

DASH Diet Food Groups

The trademark of the DASH diet in a world of diet overload, is the all encompassing and well rounded approach it takes to allowance of all major food groups. It is not limiting of any in particular, with the exception of trans fats and artificial sweetener. It is limiting only on the food groups which benefit the human body the least, being sugar, red meat, and simple carbohydrates. It is not categorized as a low carb diet, despite the modern obsession with such dieting, and it is also not quite a low calorie diet. While it does seem to emphasize less calories by portion control, if weight loss is a goal, it does not stress this point. It is mildly low fat in its approach, but it does not look at low fat in the old school method of the diet fad. Low sodium is indeed its claim to fame, as one would suspect, while attempting to lower hypertension, high blood pressure, and heart disease.

The following list of food groups allowed in this diet is based on a weight loss type of approach, and includes the necessary servings per day for an average 1600 to 3100 calorie daily intake. The findings were done by the organization who has adapted the diet at dashdiet.org. (dashdietdotorg)

WHOLE GRAINS & GRAIN PRODUCTS

- 3 CHOICES PER DAY OF WHOLE, UNPROCESSED GRAINS

The simple fact that I could not be ashamed of loving my carbs anymore made me want to start each day. I could have bagels, toast, or cereal, just as long as I would be willing to make sure that they were unprocessed and whole grain. I do love a good whole grain bagel, usually half is about right, with a tad bit of cream cheese (low fat of course) and fresh lox fish that my husband caught. It is indeed a treat washed down nicely with some orange juice.

A good lunch grain often goes handy with a whole grain wrap of choice, maybe some tuna fish and a drizzle of olive oil, salt and pepper. This is almost always a staple for lunch in my house. If wraps aren't your thing, a whole grain sandwich does the trick well, maybe with some sparkling water and a refreshing noon time treat.

Dinner time is usually my time to skimp on carbs, but if I hadn't gotten my whole serving in yet of the grains, then I would maybe treat myself to a side of brown rice or even a light Italian beer with my husband. That is an excellent summer meal pairing to a lean steak or sweet potatoes.

FRESH FRUITS

- 4-6 SERVINGS PER DAY

One thing I never could understand about the Atkins, or any of the other low carb diets was the fact that fruit was banned! This never made sense to me—and for good reason. Fruit has so much nutritional value to us as human beings, and make us feel great too. I love a grapefruit for breakfast sometimes in the summer and that alone is enough to suffice with a tiny sprinkle of sugar. Gets my day going rather well!

While fruit is very satiating for a sweet tooth, it does need to be had in moderation for the simple fact that it is not naturally abundant in all regions of the world, at all times, and it is indeed high in sugar, and that can actually do worse for someone with a weight problem, and especially Diabetes patients. I generally like to keep my fruits in the range of strawberries, blueberries, and will treat myself on occasion to higher sugar fruits like pineapple, trying to be mindful of the serving rule. It is definitely a treat to throw some frozen or fresh fruits together in a blender and make a smoothie out of them with a little almond milk or even low fat dairy of choice.

FRESH VEGGIES

- 4-6 SERVINGS PER DAY

Fresh veggies from our garden in the summer months keep me full all summer long. We grow so many varieties that I cannot name them all here. We do try to stick to our own home-grown selection, but in the off season will purchase local organic produce or buy online from a safe and reputable market. I can almost always make an entire dish out of vegetables alone. Ratatouille anyone? I also cook a mean eggplant parmesan, with a drizzle of homemade marinara, slow cooked all day on the stove top. Couldn't ask for a better and more wholesome meal; and my husband barely notices the lack of meat or fish. It is that satisfying!

Otherwise, throughout the daytime, salads are a staple in the house and a perfect treat for lunch with a homemade dressing of choice; whatever suits my mood! I often mix fruits and veggies, making scrumptious Guacamole with fresh avocado, tomato, onion and garlic which is a lip smacking treat to snack on anytime of day.

LOW FAT OR NONFAT DAIRY FOODS

- 2-4 SERVINGS PER DAY

The one main difference I notice in the DASH Diet and the Mediterranean Diet is the fact that this DASH diet allows for somewhat processed, American foods. Stuff we grew up on, like sliced American cheese, cups of yogurt, and string cheese that is kind of like Mozzarella. The fact is, we love what we love. While people living it up in bathing suits all day in the subtropical regions of Europe are eating olives and olive oil, we will take our dairy. The black and white cow thanks you kindly, as we do it. Just be sure to make sure that your dairy is either low fat or non fat, to ensure success in this diet, and limiting it to two to four times daily is enough for a couple different options throughout your day, wherever your fancy may lead you.

LEAN MEATS, FISH, POULTRY

- 1.5 TO 2.5 SERVINGS PER DAY

The meat and potatoes may not be a focal point for this diet, but it never really should be. The more I age, and the more I learn, the more I realize that our animal production for the sake of our consumption is a cause of many diseases, and even the speculation of environmental decline. The gases emitted to breed and house the livestock is atrocious. The conditions are unthinkable and I highly recommend you watch a credible documentary on the subject. It is life changing. Anyhow, because of that, I completely understand why the DASH Diet would not give us more servings of meat. If we all lived by the way of the fast food industry, we would certainly be in the condition we are now as a country. There is no need for the grease and grime of gigantic hamburgers and greasy chicken. We must be conscious in our choices of where our meat comes from and how its prepared.

Gustav and I usually eat fish, of course, and that is caught in the wild, by him. The other options for our meat consumption are strictly to have it selected from a local butcher or market where the animal is raised well and fed grass, or whatever other natural product that one animal would eat. We are especially choosy and limit our consumption of red meat to only twice per week, as a personal choice. I have found that as I make conscious decisions, knowing that we all literally "are what we eat" and the cells of that animal become us, then I am giving thanks and respect to the animal and the life that was lived. I am also rewarding and respecting my own body, which is a temple.

NUTS, SEEDS, & LEGUMES

- THREE TO SIX PER WEEK

At first glance of this nuts, seeds, and legumes category, you may, like I was, be giddy with excitement and anticipation. If you are like me, then you like snack foods. And if you are like me, you may have a weakness for bad kinds of carby snack foods, like chips and crackers. While it is a given that one must cut out those processed foods, nut and seeds, as well as legumes are a staple for health conscious dieters everywhere. But I realized quickly that the three to six suggestion was based on the week, and sadly, not to the day. But that still leaves plenty of room for safe snacking. Be very aware of the salt intake, and a serving is technically only usually a handful. Safe snacks would include unsalted almonds, sunflower seeds, and the like. I keep them handy, but not quite within arms reach of my car, my office, and my home, so that if I am ever tempted or craving snackable munchies, then I can quickly satisfy my wanting.

FATS & SWEETS

- 2 TO 4 SERVINGS PER WEEK

As a general understanding, this applies to treats like desserts and extra bonuses. In my opinion, two to four per week is a gracious allowance, as many diets won't even let you think about dessert foods for an entire phase of one or two months, or even life! That's a huge sentence. It's much more realistic and enjoyable to know I can earn my time being good, and reward myself with an icecream sundae on a hot summer day, or a slice of New York Pizza with extra cheese and pepperoni with a beer on a Friday night. It's the little indulgences that can keep us sane and also keep us in the game, coming back for more.

CHAPTER 6

PORTION CONTROL AND SERVING SIZES

As many modern diets cater to the food obsessed culture or more is more, the DASH diet may seem strict. It does emphasize a need for portion control in this bigger is better world. It does not overlook the fact that bigger is not better at all, and that quality should always remain paramount over quantity. When the diet is trying to hone in on the pandemic of hypertension, it also seems to touch on the sore subject of need for discipline and self control. The diet seems to advise against overeating, as one would think with common sense, and it advises for the use of proper and custom portion control. Each person has different needs and the will to overcome want and self sabotage is essential here.

The portion control method for the DASH Diet seems to be in the way that it breaks down specifically per person, based on age and whether male or female.

CHAPTER 7

DASH DIET FOOD LIST

The DASH Diet offers a range of foods to choose from to gain a well rounded taste and menu of choice. The lists are endless with possibilities for recipes. There are many resources online and in other books to discuss the endless ways in which food can be prepared into meals on this diet. It is certainly not a diet which you will tire from, eating the same meals over and over again.

Vegetables

Breads and Bakery Items

Cereal

Fruit

Meat, Poultry, Seafood, Soy

Grains

Dairy

Frozen Foods

Canned Goods

Condiments, Sauces, Spreads

Packaged Snacks

Nuts and Seeds

Beverages

CHAPTER 8

THE DASH DIET AND WEIGHT LOSS

While I stress the initial reason for the diet creation does not stem from the obsession in our culture for weight loss, it is a side effect which reaps the benefits due to the healthy approach in which the diet does to your body. Weight loss can be expected in this diet, as it can with many other diets. But the ultimate satisfaction to be had from the weight loss in the DASH Diet is the ability in which one will keep off the weight and maintain an optimal body image while he is practicing it.

The overused side note or fine print of *results not typical* does not apply here. If one will follow the instructions of the DASH Diet, then he or she will quickly gain success and lose weight. It is a healthy and mindful way to lose weight, which does not depend on the external implications of a supplement or trendy exercise machines. While light exercise is recommended, it is not that which causes the weight to fall off by the pound. It is indeed the nutritional value of the choices made daily in the DASH Diet which allow one to succeed.

CHAPTER 9

TIPS TO MAKE THE SWITCH TO DASH DIET EATING

As I mentioned in my introduction, the switch for me was indeed not over night. It was not within a week, but it was within the course of a year. When I say switch, it is because there is so much mental clarity needed and peace of mind with oneself to make the dedication to lifestyle changes necessary for such a feat of wellness. Especially, if one is not in a good state of mind, or health, he or she can be overwhelmed and not know just where to start. It is indeed a journey, not meant to start and stop, but to enjoy with each day as it comes. It may come with some setbacks and it probably will. But these kinds of things are to be expected and are there to help us grow. With some simple planning, and taking baby steps, it will be no time at all before you will be able to reap the benefits of the DASH Diet.

The first order of priority for the switch on taking on the DASH Diet is the need to drop expectation for overnight weight loss. It is also to realize it should not be about weight loss at all, but rather for the sake of your precious health which is your navigator in this one life. It should be a little work and a lot of joy that you come to realize this crucial element.

CHAPTER 10

TIPS TO LOWER YOUR SODIUM INTAKE

An obvious fix for sodium intake is to remove the sodas and canned goods from your life. This may be quite an easy one, but don't slip up with the canned vegetables and even diet soda. There are also a multitude of sneaky sodium sabotages in the sauces and condiments so always watch that. It's obvious also, cut out on the salt. Be aware of any processed foods, as salt and preservatives hide heavily in them.

CHAPTER 11

DASH Diet 7 Day Meal Plan

With any lifestyle change, it is utmost important to be aware of your intentions to truly change, for yourself. Unless you are lucky enough to have a personal nutritionist and a personal chef, even a live-in life coach can't quite help deter you from your own deviance. While dieting, it is very common to see people give up easily, because they slip up. If you make an intention in your head that it is not a diet and that it is a fun and creative and happy way of life, then it will be treated as such by your subconscious. It is extremely important, before you lay out the groundwork to actually make up your mind to do your best, for yourself. Because no one else is going to do it for you.

One of the tools that I find to be useful in the healthy lifestyle change is to have a course of action to put into place. For the nutritional side of things, that means making nutrition easy to accommodate, by having all of my recipes and menus planned out per week. And those recipes and menus get planned at the beginning of every week. Eventually you won't have to rely on the recipes, and then you may even feel artistic and come up with your own culinary creations, or variations of the same. If you're a minimalist, you may want to find simple and easy recipes, which keep things unfussy and less mess and stress. It is important to know what you want before you can achieve any success.

For the 7 Day Dash Diet Meal Plan, it is interesting to think on the fact that it says 7 Days. At first glimpse of Dr. Oz's approach, I wondered how that was the same as the DASH Diet I had read about elsewhere, because I knew for certain the DASH diet was not meant to last only 7 days. But perhaps, it is more of a way to organize the type of focus, mentally, that you should have regarding the diet, and to also just keep it one week at a time, so that you can be more here in the now and not worried about what you will be eating in three months. It is a way to be mindful and also keep foods fresh. With the 7 Day Diet Plan, you can really find one or two staples of meals, but then use your own creative expression to mix up the whole menu from time to time. Do what makes you happy.

CHAPTER 12

DASH MEALS – THE LIST

BREAKFAST MEALS

Apple Spiced Oatmeal

Banana Nut Pancakes

Flax Banana Yogurt Muffin

Morning Quinoa

No Bake Breakfast Granola Bars

Peanut Butter Banana Shake

Spinach Feta Mushroom Scramble

LUNCH MEALS

Apple Swiss Panini

California Grilled Sandwich

Pear Turkey Cheese Sandwich

Pita Pizza

Southwest Black Bean Cakes with Guacamole

Sunshine Wrap

Veggie Quesadillas w Cilantro Yogurt Dip

DINNER MEALS

Brown Rice Burgers

Chicken and Wild Rice Stuffed Tomatoes

Chile Rellenos

Fish Tacos

Garden Quesadillas

Mushroom Tempeh Stroganoff

Spaghetti Squash Lasagna

SNACKS

Bean Dip Athenos

Crispy Garbanzo Beans

Hummus

Potato Nachos

Skillet Granola

Tzaziki

Zucchini Pizza Bites

DESSERTS

Almond Rice Pudding

Berry Yogurt Popsicles

Cranberry Apple Risotto

Milk Chocolate Pudding

Red White & Blue Skewers

Light Pumpkin Pie

Yogurt with Fresh Strawberries & Honey

CHAPTER 13

TOP DASH Diet Recipes

APPLE SPICE BAKED OATMEAL

If you love oatmeal but you're in the mood for a change, try it baked in this recipe. Recipe courtesy of OSU Extension Service, foodhero. org.

SERVES 9

DIETITIAN'S TIP:

Add a glass of low-fat milk to make a meal that is consistent with the DASH diet guidelines. Get creative with this recipe by substituting other types of fruit for the apple. Try Oregon's state fruit, the pear, bananas, blueberries, and more.

INGREDIENTS:

1 egg, beaten

½ cup applesauce, sweetened

1 ½ cups non-fat or 1% milk

1 teaspoon vanilla

2 tablespoons oil

1 apple, chopped (about 1 ½ cups)

2 cups rolled oats

1 teaspoon baking powder

¼ teaspoon salt

1 teaspoon cinnamon

TOPPING

2 tablespoons brown sugar

2 tablespoons chopped nuts

PREPARATION:

Preheat oven to 375 degrees. Lightly oil or spray an 8 inch by 8 inch baking pan.

Combine the egg, applesauce, milk, vanilla, and oil in a bowl. Add the apple. In a separate bowl, mix the rolled oats, baking powder, salt and cinnamon. Add to the liquid ingredients and mix well. Pour mixture into baking dish and bake for 25 minutes.

Remove from oven and sprinkle with brown sugar and nuts. Return to oven and broil for 3 to 4 minutes until top is browned and the sugar bubbles. (Keep an eye on it during this step to keep it from burning).

Cut into 9, 2.5 inch by 2.5 inch squares. Serve warm. Refrigerate leftovers within 2 hours.

NUTRITION INFORMATION:

Per serving: 160 calories, 6 g total fat, 0.5 g saturated fat, 22 g carbohydrates, 6 g protein, 3 g fiber, 150 mg sodium, 69 mg calcium, 30 mg potassium, 4 mg magnesium.

BANANA NUT PANCAKES

Breakfast isn't just the most important meal anymore. With these hearty pancakes it is now the most delicious too! Recipe adopted from www.skinnytaste.com

SERVES 6

DIETITIAN'S TIP:

Forgo the syrup and top with one cup non-fat vanilla yogurt instead. The extra protein will help keep you full throughout the morning. You'll also satisfy one of three recommended dairy servings for the day.

INGREDIENTS:

1 cup whole wheat flour

2 tsp baking powder

1/4 tsp salt

1/4 tsp cinnamon

1 large banana, mashed

1 cup 1% milk

3 large egg whites

2 tsp oil

1 tsp vanilla

2 tbsp chopped walnuts

PREPARATION:

Mix all dry ingredients in a large bowl. Combine milk, egg white, oil, vanilla and mashed bananas in another bowl and mix until smooth. Combine wet ingredients with the dry and mix well with a spoon until there are no more dry spots. Don't over-mix.

Heat a large skillet on medium heat. Spray cooking spray to lightly coat griddle. Pour 1/4 cup of pancake batter onto warm griddle for each pancake. When the batter starts to bubble and the edges begin to set, flip the pancakes. Repeat with the remainder of the batter.

NUTRITION INFORMATION:

Per serving: 146 calories, 4 g total fat, 1 g saturated fat, 22 g carbohydrates, 7 g protein, 3 g fiber, 331 mg sodium, 201 mg potassium, 39 mg magnesium, 95 mg calcium

FLAX BANANA YOGURT MUFFINS

Try these muffins for a filling and fast breakfast.
Recipe courtesy of Hillary Lawson, OSU dietetic intern.

SERVES 12

DIETITIAN'S TIP:

Nutrient-rich muffins are handy for quick breakfast. Boost protein and calcium by eating muffins with a cup of yogurt or a glass of milk.

INGREDIENTS:

1 cup whole wheat flour

1 cup old-fashioned rolled oats

1 teaspoon baking soda

2 tablespoon ground flaxseed

3 large bananas, mashed (~1.5 cups)

½ cup plain, 0% fat greek yogurt

¼ cup unsweetened applesauce

¼ cup brown sugar

2 teaspoon vanilla extract

PREPARATION:

Preheat the oven to 355 degrees Fahrenheit

2) Prep the muffin tin with either cupcake liners or cooking spray.

3) Mix the dry ingredients in one bowl (flour, oats, soda, flaxseed).

4) Mix the wet ingredients in a separate bowl (banana, yogurt, applesauce, sugar, and vanilla)

5) Mix the dry ingredients into the wet ingredients until just combined. Batter should be lumpy. Do not over mix.

6) Bake for 20 to 25 minutes or until a toothpick inserted into the center of a muffin comes out with crumbs, not batter.

NUTRITION INFORMATION:

Per serving: 120 calories, 1 g total fat, 0 g saturated fat, 24 g carbohydrates, 5 g protein, 3 g fiber, 115 mg sodium, 170 mg potassium, 22 mg magnesium, 30 mg calcium

MORNING QUINOA

A rich and creamy alternative to everyday oatmeal. Recipe courtesy of Oregon State University Dietetic Intern Julie Thomas, MS

SERVES 4

DIETITIAN'S TIP:

This one-dish breakfast is gluten free and a great source of protein and calcium. Add extra milk for a thinner consistency and extra calcium!

INGREDIENTS:

2 cups low fat or nonfat milk

1 cup uncooked quinoa

¼ cup honey or brown sugar

¼ teaspoon cinnamon, plus more to taste

¼ cup sliced or slivered almonds

¼ cup dried currants, chopped dried apricots, or fresh berries

PREPARATION:

Rinse the quinoa thoroughly. Bring the milk to a boil in a medium saucepan. Add the quinoa and return to a boil. Cover, reduce heat to medium-low, and simmer until most of the liquid is absorbed (about 12-15 minutes). Remove from heat and fluff with a fork. Stir in remaining ingredients, cover, and let stand for 15 minutes.

Serving size: about 1 cup

NUTRITION INFORMATION:

320 calories, 5 g total fat, 0.5 g saturated fat, 59 g carbohydrates, 12 g protein, 4 g fiber, 70 mg sodium, 290 mg potassium, 96 mg magnesium, 172 mg calcium

NO BAKE BREAKFAST GRANOLA BARS

Take breakfast on the run with these quick and easy no bake breakfast bars. Recipe courtesy ofOregon State.

SERVES 18

DIETITIAN'S TIP:

Pack with a 1 cup container of yogurt and a piece of fruit to make it a portable meal.

INGREDIENTS:

2 1/2 cups toasted rice cereal

2 cups old fashioned oatmeal

1/2 cup raisins

1/2 cup firmly packed brown sugar

1/2 cup light corn syrup

1/2 cup peanut butter

1 teaspoon vanilla

PREPARATION:

Combine rice cereal, oatmeal, and raisins in a large mixing bowl and stir together with a wooden spoon.

In a 1-quart saucepan, mix together brown sugar and corn syrup. Turn the heat to medium-high. Stir constantly whilethe mixture is brought to a boil. Once boiling, remove the saucepan from the heat.

Stir the peanut butter and vanilla into the sugar mixture in the saucepan. Blend until smooth.

Pour the peanut butter mixture over the cereal and raisins in the mixing bowl. Mix well.

Press the mixture into a 9 x 13 baking pan. Let cool completely and cut into 18 bars.

NUTRITION INFORMATION:

Per serving: 160 calories, 5 g total fat, 1 g saturated fat, 28 g carbohydrates, 4 g protein, 2 g fiber, 75 mg sodium, 130 mg potassium, 30 mg magnesium, 17 mg calcium

PEANUT BUTTER & BANANA BREAKFAST SMOOTHIE

SERVES 1

DIETITIAN'S TIP:

With the potassium provided by the non-fat milk and the banana in this simple breakfast, this recipe is a DASH Diet dream!

INGREDIENTS:

1 cup nonfat milk

1 tablespoon all natural peanut butter

1 medium banana, frozen or fresh

PREPARATION:

Combine all ingredients in blender, and blend until very smooth.

NUTRITION INFORMATION:

Per serving: 285 calories, 8.4 g total fat, 1 g saturated fat, 42 g carbohydrates, 13 g protein, 4 g fiber, 186 mg sodium, 882 mg potassium, 32 mg magnesium, 506 mg calcium

SPINACH, MUSHROOM, AND FETA CHEESE SCRAMBLE

Get your protein and veggies in a few minutes with this simple and fresh scramble.

SERVES 1

DIETITIAN'S TIP:

This recipe is an easy way to add some fresh vegetables to your day. Get creative and throw in some fresh bell peppers, green onions, or tomatoes. You can also try using fresh grated Parmesan cheese instead of feta.

INGREDIENTS:

Cooking spray

½ cup fresh mushrooms, sliced

1 cup fresh spinach, chopped

1 whole egg and 2 egg whites

2 tablespoons feta cheese

Pepper to taste

PREPARATION:

Heat an 8-inch non-stick sauté pan over medium heat. Spray with cooking spray and add mushrooms and spinach. Sauté mushrooms and spinach for 2-3 minutes or until the spinach has wilted.

Whisk the egg and egg whites in a bowl with feta cheese and pepper if desired. Pour egg mixture over vegetables in the pan. Continue to cook eggs while stirring with a spatula for another 3-4 minutes or until the eggs are cooked through.

NUTRITION INFORMATION:

Per Serving: 150 calories, 7 g total fat, 3 g saturated fat, 6 g carbohydrate, 17 g protein, 1.5 g fiber, 441 mg sodium, 221 mg potassium, 8 mg magnesium, 95 mg calcium

LUNCH

APPLE-SWISS PANINI

This mouthwatering sandwich combines the unique tastes of Swiss cheese and arugula with the sweet crunch of sliced apples. Recipe adapted from Washington Apple Commission http://www.bestapples.com/recipes/recipe.NEW.asp?ID=284

SERVES 4

DIETITIAN'S TIP:

This sandwich would also be tasty with reduced-fat cheddar cheese. If you don't happen to have arugula handy, use fresh spinach or leaf lettuce. Enjoy with a glass of fat-free milk.

INGREDIENTS:

8 slices whole-grain bread

¼ cup non-fat honey mustard

2 crisp apples, thinly sliced

6 ounces low-fat Swiss cheese, thinly sliced

1 cup arugula leaves

Cooking spray

PREPARATION:

Preheat panini press on medium heat. If you don't have a panini press, just use a non-stick skillet.

Lightly spread honey mustard evenly over each slice of bread. Layer apple slices, cheese, and arugula leaves over 4 slices of bread. Top each with remaining bread slices.

Lightly coat panini press with cooking spray. Grill each sandwich for 3 to 5 minutes or until cheese has melted and bread has toasted. Remove from pan and allow to cool slightly before serving.

NUTRITION INFORMATION:

Per serving: 280 calories, 4.5 g total fat, 2 g saturated fat, 44 g carbohydrate, 17 g protein, 5 g fiber, 480 mg sodium, 288 mg potassium, 53 mg magnesium, 458 mg calcium.

CALIFORNIA GRILLED VEGGIE SANDWICH

Try a taste of California even meat-lovers will rave about!

Recipe adapted from MealsMatter.org

http://www.mealsmatter.org/recipes-meals/recipe/16283

SERVES 4

DIETITIAN'S TIP:

Enjoy this sandwich with a side of low-fat yogurt topped with frozen berries would to provide even more DASH foods.

INGREDIENTS:

3 tablespoons light mayonnaise

3 cloves garlic, minced

1 tablespoon lemon juice

1/8 cup olive oil

1 cup red bell peppers, sliced

1 small zucchini, sliced

1 red onion, sliced

1 small yellow squash, sliced

2 slices focaccia bread

½ cup crumbled reduced-fat feta cheese

PREPARATION:

In a bowl, mix the mayonnaise, minced garlic, and lemon juice. Set aside in the refrigerator.

Preheat the grill for high heat.

Brush vegetables with olive oil on each side. Brush grate of grill with oil. Place bell peppers and zucchini closest to middle of grill, and set onion and squash pieces around them. Cook for about 3 minutes, turn, and cook for another 3 minutes. The peppers may take a bit longer. Remove from grill and set aside.

Spread some of the mayonnaise mixture on cut sides of bread; sprinkle each with feta cheese. Place on the grill, cheese side up, and cover with lid for 2 to 3 minutes. Watch carefully so the bottoms don't burn.

Remove bread from grill and layer with vegetables. Enjoy as open faced grilled sandwiches.

NUTRITION INFORMATION:

Per serving: 240 calories, 14 g total fat, 3 g saturated fat, 24 g carbohydrate, 7 g protein, 2 g fiber, 490 mg sodium, 226 mg potassium, 11 mg magnesium, 75 mg calcium.

PEAR, TURKEY AND CHEESE SANDWICH

Fresh pear adds a gourmet touch to this easy open-faced sandwich. Recipe courtesy of USA Pears

SERVES 2

DIETITIAN'S TIP:

Some deli meats are loaded with salt, so shop carefully. When shopping for lean deli meats, look for products that are reduced sodium or low sodium. Be sure to balance a dish that contains higher amounts of sodium with accompaniments that are salt-free. Turn this sandwich into a DASH meal with a bunch of fresh grapes, cucumber slices, and fresh snap peas.

INGREDIENTS:

2 slices multi-grain or rye sandwich bread

2 tsp Dijon-style mustard

2 slices (1 oz. each) reduced-sodium cooked or smoked turkey

1 USA pear, cored and thinly sliced

1/4 cup shredded lowfat mozzarella cheese

Coarsely ground pepper

PREPARATION:

Spread each slice of bread with 1 teaspoon mustard. Place one slice turkey on each slice of bread. Arrange pear slices on turkey and sprinkle each with 2 tablespoons cheese. Sprinkle with pepper.

Broil, 4 to 6 inches from heat, 2 to 3 minutes or until turkey and pears are warm and cheese melts. Cut each sandwich in half and serve open face.

NUTRITION INFORMATION:

Per serving: 190 calories, 4 g total fat, 2 g saturated fat, 28 g carbohydrate, 13 g protein, 7 g fiber, 480 mg sodium, 268 mg calcium

PIZZA IN A PITA

This spin on a mealtime favorite is sure to have your whole family smiling!

Recipe courtesy of MealsMatter.org

http://www.mealsmatter.org/recipes-meals/recipe/15912

SERVES 2

DIETITIAN'S TIP:

Pair this meal with fresh salad greens topped with walnuts, sliced pears, and light vinaigrette.

INGREDIENTS:

2 pieces whole wheat pita bread

½ cup grated reduced sodium mozzarella cheese

¼ cup pizza or tomato sauce

Veggies of choice: mushrooms, bell pepper, onion, olives, artichoke hearts, etc

PREPARATION:

Preheat oven or toaster oven to 350 degrees. Split the pita bread halfway around the edge and spoon in the cheese, tomato sauce, and any toppings.

Wrap the pita in aluminum foil and bake for 7 to 10 minutes or until cheese melts.

NUTRITION INFORMATION:

Per serving: 170 calories, 6 g total fat, 3 g saturated fat, 21 g carbohydrate, 12 g protein, 3 g fiber, 300 mg sodium, 307 mg potassium, 36 mg magnesium, 222 mg calcium.

SOUTHWESTERN BLACK BEAN CAKES WITH GUACAMOLE

These flavorful patties taste great served with your favorite salsa and are perfect for lunch or dinner.

Recipe courtesy of MealsMatter.org

http://www.mealsmatter.org/recipes-meals/recipe/16467

SERVES 4

DIETITIAN'S TIP:

This dish is a fiber-lover's dream come true! Make it a balanced dinner with a cold glass of low fat or nonfat milk.

INGREDIENTS:

2 slices whole wheat bread, torn

3 tablespoons fresh cilantro

2 cloves garlic

1 (15-ounce) can low sodium black beans, rinsed and drained

1 (7-ounce) can chipotle peppers in adobo sauce

1 teaspoon ground cumin

1 large egg

½ medium avocado, seeded and peeled

1 tablespoon lime juice

1 small plum tomato

PREPARATION:

Place torn bread in food processor bowl or blender container. Cover and process or blend until bread resembles coarse crumbs. Transfer crumbs to a large bowl and set aside.

Process or blend cilantro and garlic until finely chopped. Add beans, 1 of the chipotle peppers, 1 to 2 teaspoons of adobo sauce, and cumin. Process or blend using on/off pulses until beans are coarsely chopped and mixture begins to pull away from sides.

Add mixture to bread crumbs in bowl. Add egg and mix well.

Shape mixture into four ½-inch-thick patties. Grill on lightly greased rack of uncovered grill directly over medium heat for 8 to 10 minutes or until patties are heated through, turning once.

Meanwhile, for guacamole, in small bowl mash avocado. Stir in lime juice. Season with salt and pepper. Serve patties with guacamole and tomato.

NUTRITION INFORMATION:

Per serving: 170 calories, 6 g total fat, 1 g saturated fat, 27 g carbohydrate, 8 g protein, 10 g fiber, 300 mg sodium, 427 mg potassium, 11 mg magnesium.

SUNSHINE WRAP

You'll be pleased at the combination of colors and flavors this rolled-up salad offers!

Recipe adapted from www.foodhero.org

SERVES 4

DIETITIAN'S TIP:

For variety, try grape halves or diced apples instead of mandarin oranges. For a meatless version, use cooked and drained garbanzo beans or tofu in place of the chicken. Adding a glass of low-fat or non-fat milk will include all food groups in this meal.

INGREDIENTS:

8 oz chicken breast (one large breast)

½ cup celery, diced

2/3 cup canned mandarin oranges, drained

¼ cup onion, minced

2 tablespoons mayonnaise

1 teaspoon soy sauce

¼ teaspoon garlic powder

¼ teaspoon black pepper

1 large whole wheat tortilla

4 large lettuce leaves, washed and patted dry

PREPARATION:

In a non-stick pan, cook chicken breast on medium-high heat until done throughout (internal temperature of 165°F). When chicken has cooled enough to handle, cut into ½ inch cubes. In medium bowl, mix chicken, celery, oranges and onions. Add mayonnaise, soy sauce, garlic and pepper. Mix gently until chicken mixture is evenly coated. Lay tortilla on clean cutting board or large plate. With a knife or clean kitchen scissors cut tortilla into four quarters. Place 1 lettuce leaf on each tortilla quarter, trimming the leaf so it doesn't hang over the tortilla. Put ¼ of the chicken mixture in the middle of each lettuce leaf. Roll tortillas up into a cone, with the two straight edges coming together and the curved edge creating the opening of the cone. Eat like a sandwich wrap. Refrigerate leftovers within 2 hours.

NUTRITION INFORMATION:

Per serving: 192 calories, 5 g total fat, 1.0 g saturated fat, 20 g carbohydrates, 16 g protein, 3 g fiber, 376 mg sodium, 349 g potassium, 24 g magnesium, 50 mg calcium

VEGGIE QUESADILLAS WITH CILANTRO YOGURT DIP

Quesadillas are a quick and easy lunch option that kids and adults enjoy. Serve them with the cilantro yogurt dip to make your meal even more festive and healthy. Make a salad of fresh in-season fruits for dessert.

Recipe adapted from www.foodhero.org

SERVES 4

DIETITIAN'S TIP:

The beans in this quesadilla are a great source of filling lean protein and dietary fiber. Corn tortillas are also a great fiber-full whole grain choice. The cilantro yogurt dip adds more flavor, protein, and calcium without adding excess calories. This meal is a great way to follow the DASH diet guidelines.

INGREDIENTS:

1 cup beans, black or pinto

2 Tablespoons cilantro, chopped

½ bell pepper, finely chopped

½ cup corn kernels

1 cup low-fat shredded cheese

6 soft corn tortillas

1 medium carrot, shredded

½ jalapeno pepper, finely minced (optional)

CILANTRO YOGURT DIP

1 cup plain non-fat yogurt

2 Tablespoons cilantro, finely chopped

Juice from ½ of a lime

PREPARATION:

Preheat large skillet over low heat.

Line up 3 tortillas. Divide cheese, corn, beans, cilantro, shredded carrots, and peppers between the tortillas. Cover each with a second tortilla.

Place a tortilla on a dry skillet and warm until cheese is melted and tortilla is slightly golden, about 3 minutes.

Flip and cook other side until golden, about 1 minute.

In a small bowl mix together the nonfat yogurt, cilantro and lime juice.

Cut each quesadilla into 4 wedges (12 wedges total) and serve 3 wedges per person with about ¼ cup of the dip.

Refrigerate leftovers within 2 hours.

NUTRITION INFORMATION:

Serving size: 3 wedges

Per serving: 240 calories, 2 g total fat, 0 g saturated fat, 42 g carbohydrates, 17 g protein, 433 mg sodium, 294 mg potassium, 9 mg magnesium, 388 mg calcium

DINNER MEALS

BROWN RICE BURGERS

The hearty flavors of this meatless burger will satisfy the meat lovers in any family.

Recipe courtesy of Bob's Red Mill

MAKES 12 BURGERS

DIETITIAN'S TIP:

Make this a DASH meal with a whole wheat bun, thick sliced tomato and sweet onion, lettuce leaf and a smear of Dijon mustard. These burgers are great with grilled or sautéed fresh asparagus spiked with garlic and olive oil. This recipe makes many burgers. Reduce the recipe by half or freeze remaining cooked burgers for a quick meal another day.

INGREDIENTS:

2 cups cooked brown rice

½ cup parsley, chopped

1 cup carrot, finely grated

½ cup onion, finely chopped

1 clove garlic, minced

1 tsp salt

¼ tsp ground black pepper

2 eggs, beaten

½ cup whole wheat flour

2 tbsp vegetable oil for cooking

PREPARATION:

Combine all ingredients except the oil in a medium mixing bowl. Form mixture into 12 patties, pressing firmly with hands.

Add vegetable oil to a skillet and heat over medium heat. Cook patties in oil until brown (4-5 minutes per side), turning only once.

NUTRITION INFORMATION:

Per burger: 120 calories, 3.5 g fat, 0 g sat fat, 18 g carbohydrate, 3 g protein, 3 g fiber, 150 mg sodium

CHICKEN AND WILD RICE STUFFED TOMATOES

Ripe tomatoes stuffed with savory chicken, wild rice, basil and parmesan cheese make a great addition to a DASH meal. Recipe Courtesy of Bailey Peterka

SERVES 4

DIETITIAN'S TIP:

Cooking rice in low-sodium broth lends great flavor to any kind of rice dish. Serve these stuffed tomatoes warm with toasted whole wheat artisan bread, or they can be prepared without the chicken making a great side dish for grilled meat.

INGREDIENTS:

1 cup uncooked wild rice (will yield 2-2 ½ cups cooked rice)
1 cup low sodium vegetable broth

1 cup water

1 chicken breast

4 large red tomatoes

2 tablespoons fresh basil

2 cloves garlic, minced

½ cup shredded parmesan cheese

2 tablespoons olive oil

PREPARATION:

Cook the wild rice according to package directions, using 1 cup of the low-sodium vegetable broth and 1 cup water (or more as package indicates) to cook rice.

Preheat the oven to 350 degrees. Grill the chicken breast and slice into 1/2" thick pieces.

Cut the top off each tomato and scoop out the insides, leaving a ½ inch thick shell.

When the rice is cooked, mix in the chicken, basil, garlic and most of the parmesan cheese, reserving some for the top of each tomato. Stuff the tomatoes with the wild rice filling and sprinkle the top with the remaining parmesan.

Brush the outside of the tomatoes with the olive oil. Bake for 20-25 minutes.

NUTRITION INFORMATION:

Per serving: 250 calories, 11 g total fat, 3 g saturated fat, 23 g carbohydrates, 14 g protein, 2 g fiber, 230 mg sodium, 172 mg potassium, 40 mg magnesium, 148 mg calcium

CHILI RELLENOS REVAMPED

A delicious and cheesy Mexican treat that fits into the DASH diet! Recipe adapted Ashley Klees of Healthy, Easy, Yum.

SERVES 6

DIETITIAN'S TIP:

Cheesy Mexican food doesn't always have to be unhealthy! In this recipe fat and calories are removed by replacing sour cream with Greek yogurt, using reduced-fat cheese, and replacing egg with avocado. Bell peppers boost nutritional content while also serving as containers for filling!

INGREDIENTS:

3 large bell peppers, any color, halved

2 eggs

4 tablespoons mashed avocado

1 1/2 cups reduced fat Mexican style cheese, shredded

1/2 cup plain non-fat Greek yogurt

1-4oz can chopped green chilies, with juice

PREPARATION:

Preheat oven to 350degrees. Wash bell peppers and cut into halves. Remove the core from peppers and remove seeds. Place pepper halves in a 7.5 x 11 inch baking pan; be sure they fit snuggly so that filling won't spill. Set aside.

In a large bowl, whisk remaining ingredients together until well combined. Evenly distribute mixture into each of the bell pepper halves, filling completely full without spilling out.

Carefully place pan in oven and cook for 30-45 minutes, or until cheese is golden brown, egg is fully cooked and a toothpick inserted comes out clean. Top with salsa and serve.

**Cooking times can vary depending on oven. If egg is still not cooked after 45 minutes, cover and bake for an additional 15-20 minutes.

NUTRITION INFORMATION:

Per serving: 150 calories, 9 g fat, 5 g saturated fat, 7 g carbohydrates, 10 g protein, 2 g fiber , 412 mg sodium, 133 mg potassium, 1 mg magnesium, 230 mg calcium

FISH TACOS

Tender cod and crunchy slaw are a perfect pair in these tangy tacos.

Recipe courtesy of Oregon State University Extension Service.

SERVES 8

INGREDIENTS:

Fish

2 pounds cod fillets

3 tablespoons lime juice (about 2 limes)

1 tomato, chopped

1/2 onion, chopped

3 tablespoons cilantro, chopped

1 teaspoon olive oil

1/4 teaspoon cayenne pepper (optional)

1/4 teaspoon black pepper

1/4 teaspoon salt

Slaw

2 cups red cabbage, shredded

1/2 cup green onions, chopped

3/4 cup nonfat sour cream

3/4 cup salsa

8 6-inch corn tortillas

PREPARATION:

Preheat oven to 350 degrees.

Rinse fish and place on rack in baking dish, to drain fat off fish.

Mix lime juice, tomato, onion, cilantro, olive oil, peppers, and salt and spoon on top of fillets. Cover loosely with aluminum foil to keep fish moist. Bake 15-20 minutes or until fish flakes.

Mix cabbage and onion; mix sour cream and salsa and add to cabbage mixture.

Divide fish among tortillas. Add 1/4 cup of slaw to each. Fold over and enjoy! Refrigerate leftovers within 2-3 hours.

NUTRITION INFORMATION:

Per serving: 180 calories, 2 g fat, 0 g saturated fat, 20 g carbohydrates, 21 g protein, 280 mg sodium, 3 g fiber, 80 mg calcium

GARDEN QUESADILLAS

There's no need to sacrifice taste when eating right. These quesadilla snacks pack a colorful flavor punch with multi-color peppers and fresh cilantro! Recipe courtesy of Dairy Council of California.

SERVES 5

DIETITIAN'S TIP:

Use whole-grain tortillas for added fiber, and fill your quesadilla with as many veggies as you like! Squash, zucchini, fresh corn, spinach, and kale are just a few additions to get closer to your daily 2 ½ cups of DASH vegetable servings.

INGREDIENTS:

2 small green and/or red sweet peppers, cut into thin strips

1 small red onion, cut into thin 1-inch-long strips

2 teaspoons olive oil or canola oil

½ teaspoon ground cumin

½ teaspoon chili powder

2 tablespoons fresh cilantro

1/3 cup fat free cream cheese (tub style)

5 (6 inch) flour tortillas

¼ cup salsa, if desired

PREPARATION:

In a large nonstick skillet cook sweet peppers and onion in 1 teaspoon of the oil for 3 to 5 minutes or until crisp-tender. Stir in cumin and chili powder. Cook and stir for 1 minute more. Stir in cilantro. Set vegetables aside.

Spread cream cheese over half of 1 side of each tortilla. Top with pepper mixture. Fold tortilla in half over peppers, pressing gently.

Place tortillas on an ungreased large baking sheet. Brush tortillas with the remaining oil. Bake in a 425 degree F oven for 5 minutes.

Cut each quesadilla into 4 wedges. Serve warm. If desired, top with salsa.

NUTRITION INFORMATION:

Per quesadilla: 58 calories, 2 g total fat, <1 g saturated fat, 8 g carbohydrate, 2 g protein, 51 mg sodium, 1 g fiber, 151 g potassium, 12 mg magnesium, 57 mg calcium

MUSHROOM TEMPEH STROGANOFF

Rich, velvety and tangy. This flavorful entrée is easy to make and tastes amazing! Try this decadent dish once, and it will become a favorite! Recipe courtesy of: http://www.wholefoodsmarket.com.

SERVES 4

DIETITIAN'S TIP:

Tempeh is a soybean product that has a nutty taste and crunchy texture. The DASH Diet recommends eating up to 6 ounces of lean protein per day. Tempeh is protein and nutrient-rich, and the tangy sour cream adds additional protein and essential vitamins and minerals to this dish. This recipe uses flavorful and wholesome ingredients to make a winning entrée, any night.

INGREDIENTS:

- 2 cups cooked brown rice (1 cup uncooked)
- 1 tablespoon canola oil
- 1 (8-ounce) package wild rice tempeh, cut into 1/2-inch thick strips
- 1/2 yellow onion, thinly sliced
- 2 cloves garlic, finely chopped
- 1 teaspoon toasted sesame oil
- 1 large Portobello mushroom, stemmed and sliced
- 1 tablespoon low sodium Worcestershire sauce
- 1 packet mushroom gravy mix
- 4 ounces non-fat sour cream
- 2 tablespoons chopped parsley

PREPARATION:

To cook brown rice, combine 1 cup uncooked brown rice and 2 cups of water in a medium saucepan. Bring mixture to a boil and then reduce to a simmer for 20 minutes, or until rice is done cooking.

Heat canola oil in a large skillet over medium heat. Add tempeh strips and cook, turning once, until both sides are golden brown. Remove tempeh from skillet and set aside. Add onions and garlic to skillet and cook until golden. Stir in sesame oil, mushrooms and

Worcestershire sauce and cook until mushrooms are soft. Return tempeh to skillet. In a measuring cup, combine gravy mix with amount of water called for on packaged directions, then stir into tempeh mixture and heat until thick. Stir in sour cream and heat just until warm. Serve stroganoff over rice, garnish with parsley.

NUTRITION INFORMATION:

Per serving: 300 calories, 8 g total fat, 1 g saturated fat, 46 g carbohydrate, 12 g protein, 6 g fiber, 410 mg sodium, 205 mg potassium, 47 mg magnesium, 163 mg calcium.

SPAGHETTI SQUASH LASAGNA

A classic recipe gets a nutritious, seasonal makeover without sacrificing flavor.

Recipe adopted from www.skinnytaste.com

SERVES 4

DIETITIAN'S TIP:

Make it a meal by adding a layer of chopped spinach, broccoli, zucchini, or any of your favorite veggies. Steam or lightly sauté veggies in a non-stick skillet until just barely tender (do not overcook) to release water before adding to lasagna. Veggies will bulk up lasagna with nutrients instead of calories.

INGREDIENTS:

2 cups marinara sauce

3 cups roasted spaghetti squash (1 large spaghetti squash)

1 cup part-skim ricotta

8 teaspoons grated parmesan cheese

6 ounces part-skim shredded mozzarella

Crushed red pepper or ground pepper to taste

PREPARATION:

To roast spaghetti squash: Cut the squash in half lengthwise, scoop out the seeds and fibers with a spoon. Place on a baking sheet, cut side up, and sprinkle with salt and pepper. Bake at 350 degrees for about an hour, or until the skin gives easily under pressure and the inside is tender. Remove from oven and let it cool 10 minutes. Using a fork, scrape out the squash flesh a little at a time. It will separate into spaghetti-like strands. Measure 3 cups for lasagna recipe. Drain off any excess liquid.

Preheat oven to 375 degrees. Spread 1 cup of marinara sauce onto bottom of baking dish. Top evenly with roasted spaghetti squash. Next, layer the ricotta cheese and sprinkle with half of the parmesan and mozzarella. Add the remaining sauce and finish with the remaining parmesan and mozzarella. Sprinkle with pepper.

Cover with foil and bake for 15-20 minutes, or until the cheese is melted and the edges begin to bubble; uncover and cook an additional 5 minutes.

NUTRITION INFORMATION:

Per serving: 291 calories, 14 g total fat, 8 g saturated fat, 21 g carbohydrates, 20 g protein, 3 g fiber, 358 mg sodium, 80 mg potassium, 8 mg magnesium, 948 mg calcium

SNACKS

BEAN DIP ATHENOS

Balsamic vinegar adds a kick to this quick, Greek-inspired bean dip. Recipe courtesy of US Dry Bean Council

SERVES 24

DIETITIAN'S TIP:

Bean-based dips and spreads help you get your DASH eating plan servings of beans, nuts and seeds. Serve this flavorful with whole grain crackers and vegetables for dipping and dunking, or spread on sandwiches. Bring two dips to the party and pair with Tzatziki, another Mediterranean style dip.

INGREDIENTS:

2 15-ounce cans, rinsed and drained, or 3 1/2 cups cooked garbanzo or navy beans

2/3 cup fat-free sour cream

2 tsp minced garlic

4 tbsp balsamic vinegar

1/4 cup chopped sun-dried tomatoes (not in oil)

1/4 cup finely chopped fresh or dried parsley

2 tbsp chopped Kalamata or ripe olives

Kalamata olives, as garnish

Assorted vegetables and crackers for serving

PREPARATION:

In the bowl of a food processor blend the beans, sour cream, garlic, and vinegar until smooth; stir in sundried tomatoes, parsley, and chopped olives.

Place the mix in a serving bowl and garnish with olives. Serve with assorted vegetables and crackers for dipping.

Dip can be made ahead of time and refrigerated overnight or for 2 to 3 hours to allow flavors to blend.

NUTRITION INFORMATION:

Per serving (2 tablespoons): 54 calories, 1 g fat, 10 g carbohydrates, 2 g protein, 2 g fiber, 100 mg sodium.

CRISPY GARBANZO BEANS

Grab a handful of these crispy garbanzo beans for a super seasoned snack. Recipe courtesy of Foodhero.org.

SERVES 8

DIETITIAN'S TIP:

Garbanzo beans are a good protein source full of heart-healthy fiber, vitamins, and minerals. Pair with some whole grain crackers, carrot sticks, or low-fat cheese for a hearty and satisfying snack. Or try them over a salad for crunchy surprise.

INGREDIENTS:

2 cans (15 ounces) unsalted garbanzo beans

½ teaspoon salt

½ teaspoon pepper

1 teaspoon garlic powder or 4 cloves of garlic

1 teaspoon onion powder

1 teaspoon dried parsley flakes

2 teaspoon dried dill

Cooking spray

PREPARATION:

Preheat oven to 400 degrees F.

Drain and rinse the garbanzo beans in a strainer. Shake off extra water. Dry the beans well with a towel to prevent "popping" in the oven.

Mix together salt, pepper, garlic powder, onion powder, parsley, and dill in a small bowl.

Lightly spray a rimmed baking sheet with cooking spray. Spread garbanzo beans onto baking sheet and lightly spray the beans with cooking spray.

Sprinkle seasoning mix over the beans and shake the pan to help distribute the seasoning. Spread the garbanzo beans into one even layer.

Place the pan on the lowest rack in the oven. Cook for 30-40 minutes, gently shaking and rotating the pan every 10-15 minutes.

The beans are done when crispy and golden brown. Let cool before serving.

NUTRITION INFORMATION:

Per serving: 111 calories, 1 g total fat, 0 g saturated fat, 20 g carbohydrates, 6 g protein, 4 g fiber, 171 mg sodium, 222 mg potassium, 35 mg magnesium, 51 mg calcium

HUMMUS

Why buy hummus when it's so easy to make? Keep this hummus on hand for convenient DASH snacking. Recipe courtesy of the US Dry Beans Council

MAKES 1 1/2 CUPS

DIETITIAN'S TIP:

Make a batch on Sunday to keep on hand in the refrigerator through the week. Hummus is chock full of garbanzo beans and Mediterranean flavors. Smear some hummus on wide strips of fresh bell peppers and wedges of whole wheat pita for a DASH snack in a flash.

INGREDIENTS:

1/3 cup toasted sesame seeds or ¼ cup tahini

1/8 tsp crushed red chilies

1 15-ounce can garbanzo beans, rinsed and drained, or 2 cups cooked garbanzo beans

1/8 cup lime, lemon or orange juice

½ tsp garlic, minced

½ tsp salt

2 tbsp olive oil

PREPARATION:

To toast sesame seeds preheat oven at 350 degrees, sprinkle sesame seeds on a baking sheet and toast for 8 to 12 minutes until golden brown, stirring frequently.

In a food processor, puree sesame seeds or tahini and chilies, then add the beans and puree. Add citrus juice, garlic and salt, puree until smooth. Finally, add oil and process until well blended. Spoon hummus into a serving bowl, cover and let stand for 1 hour to blend flavors.

NUTRITION INFORMATION:

Per serving (2 tablespoons): 39 calories, 2 g total fat, 4 g carbohydrates, 1 g protein, 47 mg sodium, 1 g fiber

POTATO NACHOS

Hosting a football party or watching the game with friends? This healthy spin on the popular nacho dish is sure to be a hit!! Recipe courtesy of Oregon State University's Food Hero https://www.foodhero.org/recipes/potato-nachos

SERVES 5

DIETITIAN'S TIP:

Using potatoes and lean ground turkey for nachos saves calories, sodium, and fat without compromising flavor. Before serving, add fat free sour cream as a final touch. Give this tasty recipe a fiber and potassium boost by substituting sweet potatoes or yams for the red potatoes. Yams are not just for Thanksgiving and fall meals. They are a great alternative to potatoes or rice in most dishes and are a great source of vitamins A and C.

INGREDIENTS:

1 pound small red potatoes, with skins on

2 teaspoons oil or cooking spray

8 ounces ground turkey, 99% fat free

½ teaspoon chili powder

½ cup cheddar cheese, shredded

1 cup lettuce, shredded

1 medium tomato, diced ¾ cup

1 cucumber, peeled and diced

1 tablespoon cilantro, chopped

¾ cup salsa

PREPARATION:

Slice potatoes into small circles about 1/4 inch thick. Lightly coat the potato slices with oil (or spray for 3 seconds with cooking spray). Arrange slices on a baking sheet in a single layer. Bake in the oven at 450 degrees for 25-30 minutes, depending on desired darkness.

Meanwhile, add ground turkey and chili powder to a skillet. Cook, stirring over medium heat for 8-10 minutes or until turkey browns. Remove potatoes from the oven. Transfer baked potatoes to a casserole dish or an oven-safe dish. Top with turkey and sprinkle with cheese. Put back in the oven to melt the cheese, about 2 minutes. Remove from oven and top with lettuce, tomato, cucumber, cilantro, and salsa. Refrigerate leftovers within 2-3 hours.

NUTRITION INFORMATION:

Per Serving: 192 calories, 6 g total fat, 3 g of carbohydrates, 16 g protein, 2 g of fiber, 242 mg sodium, 531 mg potassium, 24 mg magnesium, 19 mg calcium

SKILLET GRANOLA

An on-the-go, low-calorie treat packed with flavor!

Recipe courtesy of OSU Extension Service; foodhero.org

SERVES 24

DIETITIAN'S TIP:

Make it a parfait! Serve granola atop low-fat plain yogurt with fresh fruit to add more calcium and fiber.

INGREDIENTS:

1/3 cup vegetable oil

3 tablespoons honey

¼ cup powdered milk

1 teaspoon vanilla

4 cups uncooked, old-fashioned rolled oats

½ cup sunflower seeds

1 cup raisins

PREPARATION:

• Line a baking sheet with parchment or waxed paper.

• Warm oil and honey in a skillet for one minute over medium heat. Add powdered milk and vanilla.

• Stir in oats and sunflower seeds, and mix until coated with oil and honey mixture. Heat over medium heat. Stir until oatmeal is slightly brown.

• Take off heat. Stir in raisins. Pour granola onto lined baking sheet. Spread evenly over baking sheet.

• Cool mixture. Store in an airtight container (jar or plastic bag).

NUTRITION INFORMATION:

Per serving: 120 calories, 5 g fat, 0.5 g saturated fat, 17 g carbohydrates, 3 g protein, 2 g fiber, 5 mg sodium, 88 mg potassium, 4 mg magnesium, 14 mg calcium

TZATZIKI

Tzatziki is a cool and refreshing Greek yogurt and cucumber sauce. Use it as a dip, spread or condiment. Recipe courtesy of Carrie Weinstein.

MAKES 3 1/2 CUPS

DIETITIAN'S TIP:

The key to great tzatziki is the thick, creamy texture. For this reason, it is important to strain the yogurt well before making this sauce. Tzatziki is a delicious dip to serve with sliced vegetables like bell peppers, squash or carrots. But it also makes for a tasty accompaniment to grilled chicken or fish. For a slight variation, try adding 1 tablespoon freshly chopped mint.

INGREDIENTS:

3 cups of low-fat plain yogurt

3 tbsp lemon juice

1 garlic clove, finely minced

2 medium cucumbers, peeled and seeded

1 tbsp chopped fresh dill

½ tsp salt

¼ tsp black pepper

PREPARATION:

Place the plain yogurt in a paper towel-lined strainer and set it over a bowl. Place the bowl in the refrigerator for 2 hours so the yogurt can drain. Transfer the thickened yogurt to a large bowl.

Grate the cucumber into a small bowl and toss with ¼ teaspoon salt. Wrap the grated cucumber in paper towel and gently squeeze as much liquid from the cucumber as you can. Add the cucumber to the yogurt.

Mix in the lemon juice, garlic, dill, remaining salt, and pepper. Allow the tzatziki to sit in the refrigerator for a few hours for the flavors to blend. Serve chilled or at room temperature.

NUTRITION INFORMATION:

Per Serving (¼ cup): 37 calories, 0.5 g fat, 0.5 g saturated fat, 4 g carbohydrate, 3 g protein, 120 mg sodium, 0 g fiber, 90 mg calcium.

ZUCCHINI PIZZA BITES

This flavorful side dish satisfies your craving for pizza, without the guilt! Recipe adapted from www.skinnytaste.com

SERVES 1

DIETITIAN'S TIP:

Enjoy these pizza bites as a mid-afternoon snack. They also make a great light lunch when served with a green salad and a slice of whole-grain bread and a glass of low-fat or fat-free milk.

INGREDIENTS:

4 slices large zucchini, cut ¼ inch thick

spray olive oil (or non-stick cooking spray)

pepper

4 tablespoon pizza sauce

2 tablespoon shredded part-skim mozzarella cheese

PREPARATION:

Preheat broiler to 500°F.

Spray both sides of each zucchini slice lightly with olive oil or cooking spray and season with pepper. Place zucchini slices in the broiler for 2 minutes, turn over, and broil 2 minutes longer. Remove from broiler and top each slice with 1 tablespoon pizza sauce and ½ tablespoon cheese. Broil for an additional minute or two, until cheese is melted. Serve immediately.

NUTRITION INFORMATION:

Per serving: 69 calories, 4 g total fat, 1.7 g saturated fat, 5 g carbohydrates, 5 g protein, 1 g fiber, 136 mg sodium, 228 g potassium, 17 g magnesium, 127 mg calcium

DESSERTS

ALMOND RICE PUDDING

Go nuts over this tasty little treat!

Recipe adapted from Oregon State University's Food Hero

SERVES 6

DIETITIAN'S TIP:

Try using brown rice instead of white to for extra fiber. This yummy dessert contributes ½ cup toward your daily goal of 3 cups milk.

INGREDIENTS:

3 cups 1% milk

1 cup white rice

1⁄4 cup sugar

1 teaspoon vanilla

1⁄4 teaspoon almond extract

cinnamon to taste

1⁄4 cup toasted almonds — optional

PREPARATION:

Combine milk and rice in a medium saucepan, and bring to a boil.

Reduce heat and simmer for 1/2 hour with the lid on until the rice is soft.

Remove from heat and add the sugar, vanilla, almond extract, and cinnamon.

Sprinkle toasted almonds on top and serve warm.

Refrigerate leftovers within 2-3 hours.

NUTRITION INFORMATION:

Serving size: ½ cup
Per serving: 180 calories, 1.5 g total fat, 1 g saturated fat, 36 g carbohydrates, 7 g protein, 1 g fiber, 65 mg sodium, 1 mg potassium, 0 mg magnesium, 150 mg calcium

BERRY YOGURT POPSICLES

A refreshing, nutrient-rich treat for summer days, especially when berry season hits Oregon. Use small disposable cups or an ice cube tray with toothpicks if you don't have a popsicle mold. Adapted from www.skinnytaste.com.

SERVES 8

DIETITIAN'S TIP:

Fresh fruit popsicles are a fun and special way to entice your family to eat a wider variety of fruits! They fit perfectly into the DASH diet plan by providing fruit and low-fat dairy in a low calorie, low sugar treat that is packed with antioxidants and calcium. Experiment with other fruit and yogurt combinations to make layered popsicles; the possibilities are limitless.

INGREDIENTS:

For the purple layer:

1 cup blueberries

1 cup blackberries

1 cup non-fat or low-fat plain yogurt

1 ¼ cup non-fat or low-fat milk

PREPARATION:

Blend the ingredients in a blender.

Pour about ½ cup of the smoothie mixture into your molds or

cups. (Depending on the size of your mold you may need more or less mixture per popsicle)

Freeze for 30 minutes.

Remove from the freezer and insert the sticks then freeze them for one hour or until hard.

NUTRITION INFORMATION:

Servings: 8

Per serving: 47 calories, 0 g total fat, 0 g saturated fat, 9 g carbohydrates, 3 g protein, 1 g fiber, 43 mg sodium, 43 mg potassium, 5 mg magnesium, 102 mg calcium

CRANBERRY APPLE DESSERT RISOTTO

From Meals Matter

Risotto has become the hottest item on Italian menus, but this unique recipe is a dessert risotto, replacing the usual stock and wine with milk and fruit juice. If you like rice pudding, you'll love this!

SERVES 4

INGREDIENTS:

½ cup dried cranberries

3 ½ cups fat-free milk or 1% lowfat milk

1 cinnamon stick

1 pinch salt

1 tbsp butter

1 large golden delicious apple, peeled, cored and finely diced (1 ½ cups)

½ cup Arborio rice

1 ½ cups apple cider

2 tbsp packed light brown sugar

PREPARATION:

In a small bowl, cover dried cranberries with boiling water. Set aside for 20 to 30 minutes to plump.

Heat milk, cinnamon stick and salt on the stovetop or in microwave until steaming hot, but not boiling. Remove from the heat, cover and set aside to steep.

In a heavy, deep sauté pan or Dutch oven, heat butter over medium heat. Add apple and cook, stirring frequently, until tender, 1 to 2 minutes. Add rice and cook, stirring constantly, 30 seconds. Add 3/4 cup apple cider and cook, stirring, until most of the liquid has evaporated, 1 to 2 minutes. Add the remaining 3/4 cup of the apple cider and cook, stirring, until most of the liquid has evaporated. Add sugar and mix well.

Add 1/2 cup of the warm milk and the cinnamon stick to the rice mixture and cook, stirring frequently, until almost all of it has been absorbed, 2 to 3 minutes.

Continue cooking and stirring, adding remaining milk, 1/2 cup at a time, until the rice is tender and the risotto has a creamy consistency. Total cooking time will be about 20 minutes. Remove from the heat and discard cinnamon stick.

Drain cranberries and stir into risotto, along with vanilla. Let cool for at least 10 minutes before serving warm.

NUTRITION INFORMATION:

Per serving: 336 calories, 3.5 g total fat, 2 g saturated fat, 71 g carbohydrates, 9 g protein, 279 mg calcium, 103 mg sodium, 3 g fiber.

MILK CHOCOLATE PUDDING

Did someone say guilt-free chocolate? Here's a dessert that will satisfy your sweet tooth for under 200 calories. Recipe from Oregon Dairy Council

SERVES 4

DIETITIAN'S TIP:

Top pudding with sliced bananas or strawberries to add a serving of fruit to your dessert. You can even try sprinkling pudding with ground flaxseed for a slightly nutty flavor and a dose of omega-3 fatty acids.

INGREDIENTS:

3 tablespoons cornstarch

2 tablespoons cocoa powder

2 tablespoons sugar

1/8 teaspoon salt

2 cups nonfat milk

1/3 cup chocolate chips

1/2 teaspoon vanilla

PREPARATION:

In a medium saucepan, mix cornstarch, cocoa powder, sugar and salt until well combined. Whisk in milk. Heat over medium, stirring frequently, until thickened and just beginning to bubble. Remove from heat; stir in chocolate chips and vanilla until chocolate chips are melted and pudding is smooth.

Pour into 4 serving dishes or one large dish and chill until set. To prevent a skin from forming on top place plastic wrap on the surface of the pudding.

NUTRITION INFORMATION:

Per serving: 197 calories, 5 g total fat, 3 g saturated fat, 31 g carbohydrates, 6 g protein, 3 g fiber, 138 mg sodium, 1 mg potassium, 0 mg magnesium, 125 mg calcium

RED WHITE & BLU RED, WHITE, AND BLUE FRUIT SKEWERS WITH CHEESECAKE YOGURT DIP

These skewers make an attractive summertime dessert that kids love! Recipe courtesy ofskinnytaste.com.

SERVES 24

DIETITIAN'S TIP:

Double the fruit and halve the cake for an even lighter dessert. Substitute raspberries, red grapes, and other fruits as desired.

INGREDIENTS:

For the cheesecake dipping sauce:

4 ounces 1/3 less fat cream cheese (Neufchatel), softened

1 cup fat free Greek yogurt

1 teaspoon vanilla extract

¼ cup sugar

For the skewers:

14 ounces angel food cake, cut into 1-inch cubes

72-84 medium strawberries (about 3 ½ pounds), stems removed

1 pint blueberries

24-28 skewers

PREPARATION:

In a medium bowl, combine the cream cheese with yogurt, vanilla and sugar. Mix well until sugar dissolves. Set aside.

Thread 3 strawberries and 2 cubes of cake onto each skewer, alternating between strawberries and cake. Finish each skewer with 3 blueberries. Place finished skewers on a platter. Refrigerate skewers and dip until ready to eat.

Serving size: 1 skewer, 1 tablespoon yogurt dip

NUTRITION INFORMATION:

100 calories, 1 g total fat, 0.5 g saturated fat, 19 g carbohydrates, 3 g protein, 1 g fiber, 140 mg sodium, 109 mg potassium, 3 mg magnesium, 43 mg calcium.

THE BEST LIGHT PUMPKIN PIE RECIPE

Nothing says fall like a slice of homemade pumpkin pie. Sink your teeth into this heart healthy version of the holiday must-have dessert.

Recipe courtesy of www.mealsmatter.org

SERVES 8

DIETITIAN'S TIP:

Tis' the season to indulge in pumpkin! The fall vegetable is low in fat and calories, but high in the vitamins A and C. Pumpkin is also high in fiber, which aids digestion and contributes to a healthy heart. Try this: Heat 1 cup canned pumpkin with a drizzle of honey and a sprinkling of cinnamon, cardamom, and nutmeg for a healthy snack. Add the mixture to one serving of instant oatmeal for a complete and filling breakfast.

INGREDIENTS:

1 cup ginger snaps

16 ounces canned pumpkin

1/2 cup egg whites

1/2 cup sugar

2 teaspoons pumpkin pie spice

12 ounce can evaporated skim milk

PREPARATION:

Preheat oven to 350. Grind the cookies in a food processor. Lightly spray a 9" glass pie pan with vegetable cooking spray. Pat the cookie crumbs into the pan evenly.

Mix the rest of the ingredients in a medium-sized mixing bowl. Pour into the crust and bake until knife inserted in center comes out clean, about 45 minutes.

Store in the refrigerator. Allow to cool and slice in 8 wedges.

NUTRITION INFORMATION:

Per serving: 165 calories, 2 g total fat, 1 g saturated fat, 32 g carbohydrates, 6 g protein, 2 g fiber, 170 mg sodium, 291 mg potassium, 2 mg magnesium, 138 mg calcium

YOGURT WITH FRESH STRAWBERRIES AND HONEY

Cool, creamy yogurt with ripe strawberries is a perfect dessert on a warm summer evening.

SERVES 4

DIETITIAN'S TIP:

Fresh fruit, like ripe strawberries, are naturally sweet and require very little preparation. Try focusing your summer desserts on simple preparations of naturally sweet fresh fruit with lowfat or fat-free yogurt. This recipe is a perfect way to get your DASH servings of dairy, fruit and nuts.

INGREDIENTS:

1 pint fresh strawberries

4 teaspoons honey

3 cups plain lowfat yogurt

4 Tablespoons toasted sliced almonds

PREPARATION:

Clean and slice strawberries into quarters, set aside.

Place ¾ cup of yogurt into each of 4 serving dishes. Divide the strawberries evenly among the dishes. Top each with 1 teaspoon honey and then 1 tablespoon toasted sliced almonds. Serve immediately.

NUTRITION INFORMATION:

Per Serving: 190 calories, 5 g total fat, 2 g saturated fat, 26 g carbohydrates, 11 g protein, 2 g fiber, 130 mg sodium, 364 mg calcium

CONCLUSION

The DASH Diet is no miracle drug, and is by far the Western culture's best attempt at a holistic approach to life. It is not pushed by the Pharmaceutical Companies to gain your money, or by the celebrities to gain your attention and adoration. It is not pushed for the sake of greed by any means and is a general concern of our government for its people and the slow and gradual decline of the nation's health. It is absolutely critical that you take actions today to follow this regimen and help to spread the word to the people you love dearly, and the enemies perhaps that could use it too. The world may be a better place overall if people start to realize the food they put in their body is the best medicine that will hopefully never have a need to be prescribed. It is up to you to make the best of it.

WORKS CITED

"7-Day DASH Diet Meal Plan." 7-Day DASH Diet Meal Plan. Www.doctoroz.com, 18 Feb. 2013. Web. 12 Apr. 2015

"The DASH Diet Eating Plan." The DASH Diet for Healthy Weight Loss, Lower Blood Pressure & Cholesterol. Www.dashdiet. org, n.d. Web. 12 Apr. 2015.

My name is Valerie Childs . . .

And I love people.

My purpose in life is to help as many people as possible reach their greatest potential physically, emotionally and spiritually.

As a life coach and nutrition coach, I've have for years coached in small groups and 1 on 1 until one day I realized this is not helping the multitudes of people I dreamed of helping.

I also found I was doing people a disservice by not putting down on paper all my years of knowledge and experience about what really works when it comes to weight loss, true natural health, and the importance of loving ourselves.

My heart breaks for people with destructive patterns that slowly kill them on the inside. Patterns such as terrible eating habits, (food) addictions, people whom never stop dieting, women and men who are never satisfied with the person they see in the mirror no matter how much they improve.

You know how they say many foods are terrible for us, the so-called "silent killers". The true silent killer however is really our own self. The feeling of never being good enough.

I want to make a change in the world. To provide true information about natural health, weight loss and overall well-being.

I know that by reading and applying the weight loss strategies I have provided you with in my books, you will lose weight. You will fit into your jeans and dresses again.

But more importantly, I hope by being acquainted with me you can finally start the journey of loving yourself. That when you look yourself in the mirror you will see how beautiful you are, no matter what size or what the number on the scale says.

My hope for you is that you will start SEEING yourself, the person you, how wonderfully made you are, and that you'll discover your unique purpose in life.

I talk about all of these important subjects in my newsletter, so make sure you're signed up to receive them. (You'll also get notified when I have books out for free).

xx Valerie

CHECK OUT THESE OTHER BOOKS
FROM VALERIE CHILDS!

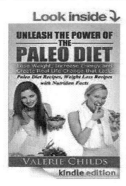

Paleo Diet: Unleash the Power of the Paleo Diet: Lose Weight, Increase Energy and Create Real Life Change That Lasts

Check it out here → http://www.amazon.com/dp/B00VAMI5PY

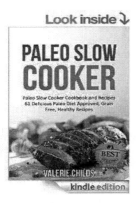

Paleo Slow Cooker: Paleo Slow Cooker Cookbook and Recipes–61 Delicious Paleo Diet Approved, Grain Free, Healthy Recipes–BONUS–Paleo Cookbook Recipes

http://www.amazon.com/dp/B00W0E1US0

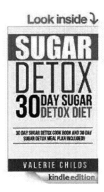

Sugar Detox: 30 Day Sugar Detox Diet–30 Day Sugar Detox Cook Book, Recipes and Meal Plan Included!

Check it out here → http://www.amazon.com/dp/B00W0G9TF4

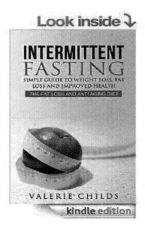

Intermittent Fasting: Simple Guide to Weight Loss, Fat Loss, and Improved Health–THE FAT LOSS AND ANTI AGING DIET

http://www.amazon.com/dp/B00VVC6O4W

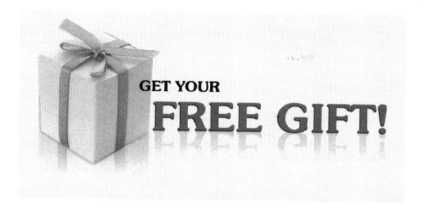

WAIT! – DO YOU LIKE FREE BOOKS?0

My **FREE Gift** to You!! As a way to say **Thank You** for downloading my book, I'd like to offer you more **FREE BOOKS!** Each time we release a NEW book, we offer it first to a small number of people as a test–drive. Because of your commitment here in downloading my book, I'd love for you to be a part of this group. You can join easily here ➔ http://rapidslimdown.com/

CONCLUSION

Thank you again for downloading this book!

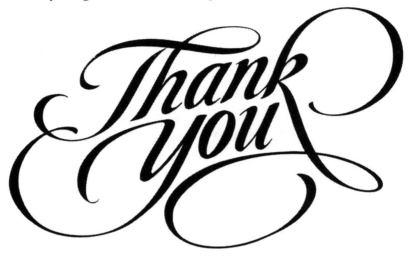

If you enjoyed this book, then I'd like to ask you for a favor, would you be kind enough to leave a review for this book on Amazon? It'd be greatly appreciated!

Help us better serve you by sending questions or comments to greatreadspublishing@gmail.com - Thank you!

Made in the USA
Columbia, SC
14 January 2018